This publication is intended to provide educational information for the reader on the covered subjects. It is not intended to take the place of personalized medical counseling, diagnosis, and treatment from a trained healthcare professional.

ISBN 978-1-998455-79-9 (Paperback)
ISBN 978-1-998455-80-5 (eBook)

Printed and bound in USA
Published by Loons Press

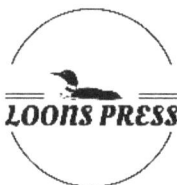

LOONS PRESS

I0096214

Table Of Contents

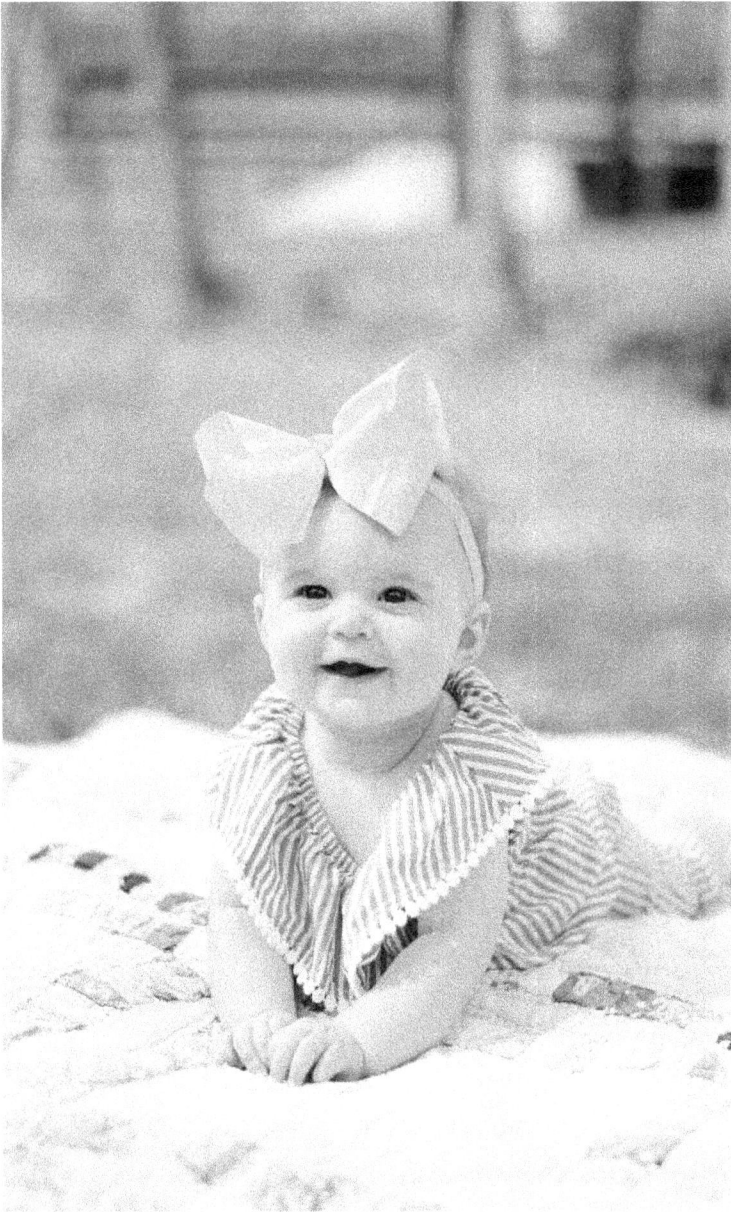

Chapter 1

Understanding RSV

What is RSV?

Respiratory Syncytial Virus (RSV) is a common virus that affects the respiratory system, particularly in young children and older adults. It is easily spread through respiratory secretions, such as coughing and sneezing, making it highly contagious.

RSV can cause symptoms similar to the common cold, such as coughing, sneezing, and a runny nose. However, in some cases, RSV can lead to more severe respiratory infections, such as bronchiolitis or pneumonia, especially in infants and elderly individuals.

Preventing RSV is crucial, especially for those who are at higher risk of developing severe complications from the virus. There are several natural solutions that can help prevent the spread of RSV.

One of the most important ways to prevent RSV is through proper hand hygiene. Washing hands frequently with soap and water, especially after coughing or sneezing, can help reduce the spread of the virus. Additionally, avoiding close contact with individuals who are sick with RSV can also help prevent its transmission.

Another natural way to prevent RSV is by maintaining a healthy immune system. Eating a well-balanced diet rich in fruits, vegetables, and whole grains can help support the immune system and reduce the risk of infections.

Regular exercise, getting an adequate amount of sleep, and managing stress levels are also important factors in maintaining a healthy immune system. In addition, staying hydrated by drinking plenty of water can help keep the respiratory system functioning properly and reduce the risk of infections.

For individuals who are at higher risk of developing severe complications from RSV, such as infants, the elderly, or individuals with underlying health conditions, there are additional steps that can be taken to prevent the virus.

One such measure is ensuring that all family members and caregivers are up to date on their vaccinations, such as the flu vaccine, as respiratory viruses like RSV can often be more severe in individuals who are already sick with another infection. In some cases, healthcare providers may recommend medications or treatments to help prevent RSV in high-risk individuals.

Overall, preventing RSV naturally is possible through simple yet effective measures such as proper hand hygiene, maintaining a healthy immune system, and avoiding close contact with individuals who are sick. By taking these steps, individuals can reduce their risk of contracting RSV and protect themselves and others from the potentially severe complications associated with the virus.

It is important for those who are concerned about RSV to be informed about the virus and the preventative measures that can be taken to reduce its spread.

Symptoms of RSV

RSV, or respiratory syncytial virus, is a common respiratory virus that can affect people of all ages, but is most dangerous for infants and older adults. Recognizing the symptoms of RSV is crucial in order to seek medical attention and prevent the spread of the virus.

Symptoms of RSV can vary depending on the age of the individual, but common signs include coughing, wheezing, fever, and difficulty breathing. It is important to be aware of these symptoms in order to take appropriate action to prevent further complications.

In infants, symptoms of RSV can be particularly severe and may include rapid breathing, irritability, poor feeding, and bluish skin color. If your infant is displaying any of these symptoms, it is important to seek medical attention immediately. Older adults may experience symptoms such as coughing, shortness of breath, and fatigue. These symptoms can be mistaken for a common cold or flu, so it is important to be vigilant and seek medical attention if necessary.

Preventing the spread of RSV is crucial in protecting vulnerable populations from the virus. One of the best ways to prevent RSV is through good hygiene practices, such as washing hands frequently and avoiding close contact with sick individuals. Additionally, staying home when sick and covering coughs and sneezes can help prevent the spread of the virus. It is important to be mindful of these preventive measures in order to protect yourself and others from RSV.

Natural solutions for preventing RSV can also be effective in reducing the risk of infection. Consuming immune-boosting foods such as fruits and vegetables, getting plenty of rest, and staying hydrated can help strengthen the immune system and prevent illness.

Additionally, using essential oils such as eucalyptus and tea tree oil can help support respiratory health and reduce congestion. By incorporating these natural solutions into your daily routine, you can help protect yourself and your loved ones from RSV.

In conclusion, being aware of the symptoms of RSV and taking proactive steps to prevent infection are crucial in protecting yourself and others from this common respiratory virus. By recognizing the signs of RSV, practicing good hygiene habits, and incorporating natural solutions into your routine, you can reduce the risk of infection and stay healthy.

Remember, prevention is key when it comes to RSV, so be sure to take the necessary precautions to protect yourself and your loved ones.

Who is at risk for RSV?

Respiratory Syncytial Virus (RSV) is a common respiratory virus that can affect people of all ages, but certain groups are at a higher risk for developing severe complications from the virus. Infants and young children, especially those under the age of 2, are among the most vulnerable to RSV. This is because their immune systems are still developing, making it harder for them to fight off the virus.

Premature babies are also at a higher risk for RSV, as their lungs are often underdeveloped and they may have other health issues that make them more susceptible to severe respiratory infections. Additionally, children with chronic lung or heart conditions, as well as those with weakened immune systems, are at an increased risk for complications from RSV.

Adults over the age of 65, especially those with underlying health conditions such as heart or lung disease, are also considered to be at a higher risk for severe complications from RSV. This is because their immune systems may not be as strong as they once were, making it more difficult for them to fight off the virus.

Pregnant women are another group that should take precautions to prevent RSV, as they are more likely to experience severe complications if they contract the virus. It is important for pregnant women to take steps to protect themselves and their unborn babies from RSV, such as avoiding close contact with sick individuals and practicing good hand hygiene.

Overall, it is important for individuals who are at a higher risk for RSV to take steps to prevent the virus, such as practicing good hand hygiene, avoiding close contact with sick individuals, and staying home when feeling unwell. By taking these precautions, individuals can reduce their risk of developing severe complications from RSV and protect their health and the health of those around them.

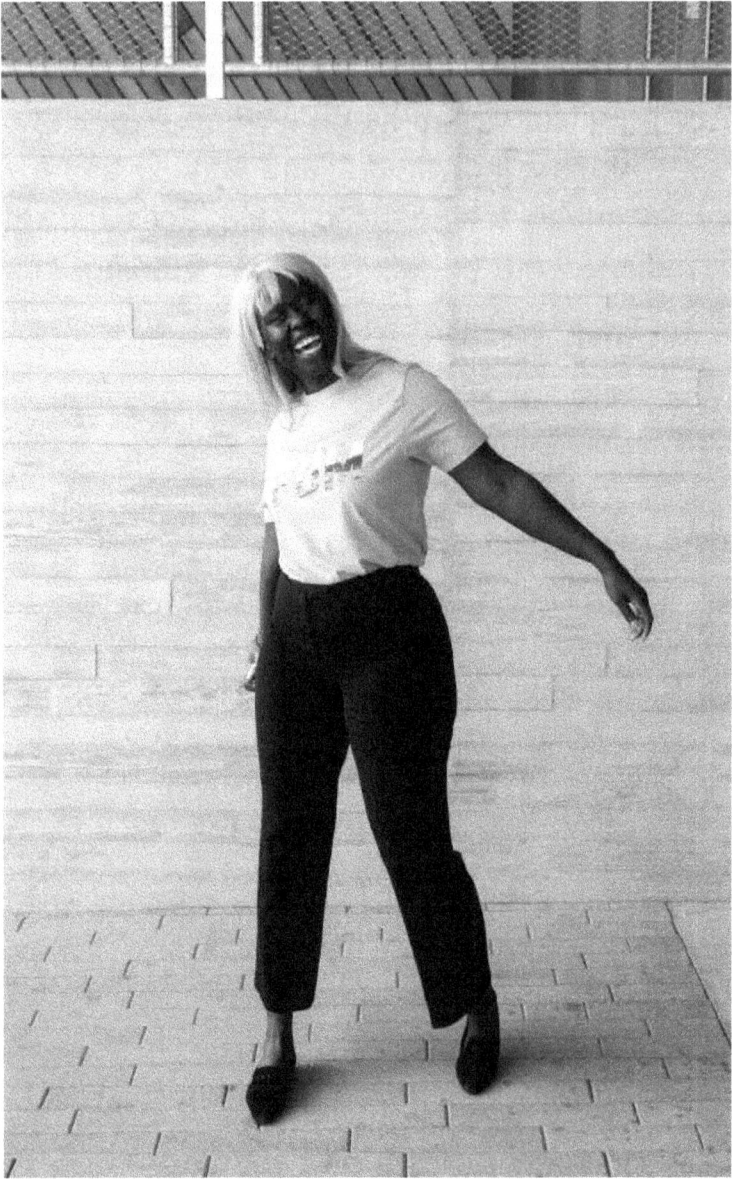

Chapter 2

Traditional Treatments for RSV

Medications for RSV

RSV, or respiratory syncytial virus, is a common respiratory virus that affects people of all ages, but can be particularly dangerous for young children and older adults. In severe cases, RSV can lead to pneumonia or bronchiolitis, so it is important to take steps to prevent the virus from spreading. While there are medications available to help treat RSV, they are typically only recommended for severe cases or for individuals with weakened immune systems.

For infants and young children with RSV, doctors may prescribe antiviral medications such as ribavirin to help reduce the severity of symptoms and prevent complications. These medications are typically given through a nebulizer or inhaler and must be closely monitored by a healthcare provider. It is important to follow the prescribed dosage and treatment schedule to ensure the medication is effective in fighting the virus.

In some cases, doctors may also recommend using bronchodilators or corticosteroids to help alleviate symptoms such as wheezing or difficulty breathing. These medications can help open up the airways and reduce inflammation in the lungs, making it easier for the individual to breathe. However, it is important to use these medications under the guidance of a healthcare provider, as they can have side effects and may not be suitable for everyone.

While medications can help treat RSV symptoms, it is important to remember that prevention is key in reducing the spread of the virus. Practicing good hygiene, such as washing hands frequently and avoiding close contact with sick individuals, can help prevent the spread of RSV.

Additionally, maintaining a healthy lifestyle, including eating a balanced diet and getting regular exercise, can help strengthen the immune system and reduce the risk of contracting RSV.

In conclusion, while medications can help treat severe cases of RSV, prevention is the best way to protect yourself and your loved ones from the virus.

By following simple steps such as practicing good hygiene and maintaining a healthy lifestyle, you can reduce your risk of contracting RSV and help keep yourself and your community healthy. If you have concerns about RSV or are experiencing severe symptoms, it is important to seek medical attention from a healthcare provider.

Hospitalization for RSV

Hospitalization for RSV can be a frightening experience for both children and their parents. Respiratory syncytial virus, or RSV, is a common virus that affects the respiratory system and can lead to serious complications, especially in young children and infants. In some cases, hospitalization may be necessary to monitor and treat the symptoms of RSV.

When a child is hospitalized for RSV, they will likely receive supportive care to help them breathe more easily and reduce the severity of their symptoms. This may include oxygen therapy, intravenous fluids, and medications to help open up the airways and reduce inflammation in the lungs. In severe cases, a child may need to be placed on a ventilator to help them breathe.

It is important for parents to follow the treatment plan outlined by healthcare providers and to ask questions if they are unsure about any aspect of their child's care. Hospitalization for RSV can be a stressful time, but knowing that your child is in good hands and receiving the necessary medical care can provide some comfort during this difficult time.

Preventing RSV is always the best course of action, and there are natural solutions that can help reduce the risk of infection. Good hygiene practices, such as washing hands frequently and avoiding close contact with sick individuals, can help prevent the spread of RSV. Additionally, keeping a clean and well-ventilated home environment can help reduce the risk of exposure to the virus.

By taking proactive steps to prevent RSV and seeking prompt medical care if symptoms develop, parents can help protect their children from the serious complications associated with this common virus. Hospitalization for RSV can be a scary experience, but with the right support and care, most children are able to recover fully and go on to lead healthy lives.

Potential side effects of traditional treatments

When it comes to preventing RSV, many people turn to traditional treatments such as antiviral medications and vaccines. While these treatments can be effective in some cases, it's important to be aware of the potential side effects that can come with them.

In this subchapter, we will explore some of the common side effects associated with traditional RSV treatments.

One potential side effect of traditional RSV treatments is gastrointestinal issues. Many antiviral medications can cause stomach upset, nausea, and diarrhea. These side effects can be especially troubling for young children who may already be struggling with feeding issues due to the virus. It's important to monitor your child's symptoms closely and consult with a healthcare provider if you notice any concerning changes in their digestive health.

Another common side effect of traditional RSV treatments is respiratory issues. Some antiviral medications can cause bronchospasms, wheezing, and difficulty breathing. This can be particularly concerning for individuals who already have underlying respiratory conditions such as asthma.

If you or your child experience any respiratory symptoms while taking traditional RSV treatments, it's important to seek medical attention immediately.

In addition to gastrointestinal and respiratory issues, traditional RSV treatments can also have neurological side effects. Some antiviral medications have been linked to headaches, dizziness, and confusion. These side effects can be particularly concerning for children, as they may not be able to communicate their symptoms effectively.

If you notice any changes in your child's behavior or cognitive function while on traditional RSV treatments, it's important to speak with a healthcare provider right away.

Overall, while traditional RSV treatments can be effective in some cases, it's important to be aware of the potential side effects that can come with them. By staying informed and monitoring your symptoms closely, you can help ensure a safe and effective treatment plan for yourself or your child. In the next chapter, we will explore some natural solutions for preventing RSV that may offer a safer and gentler alternative to traditional treatments.

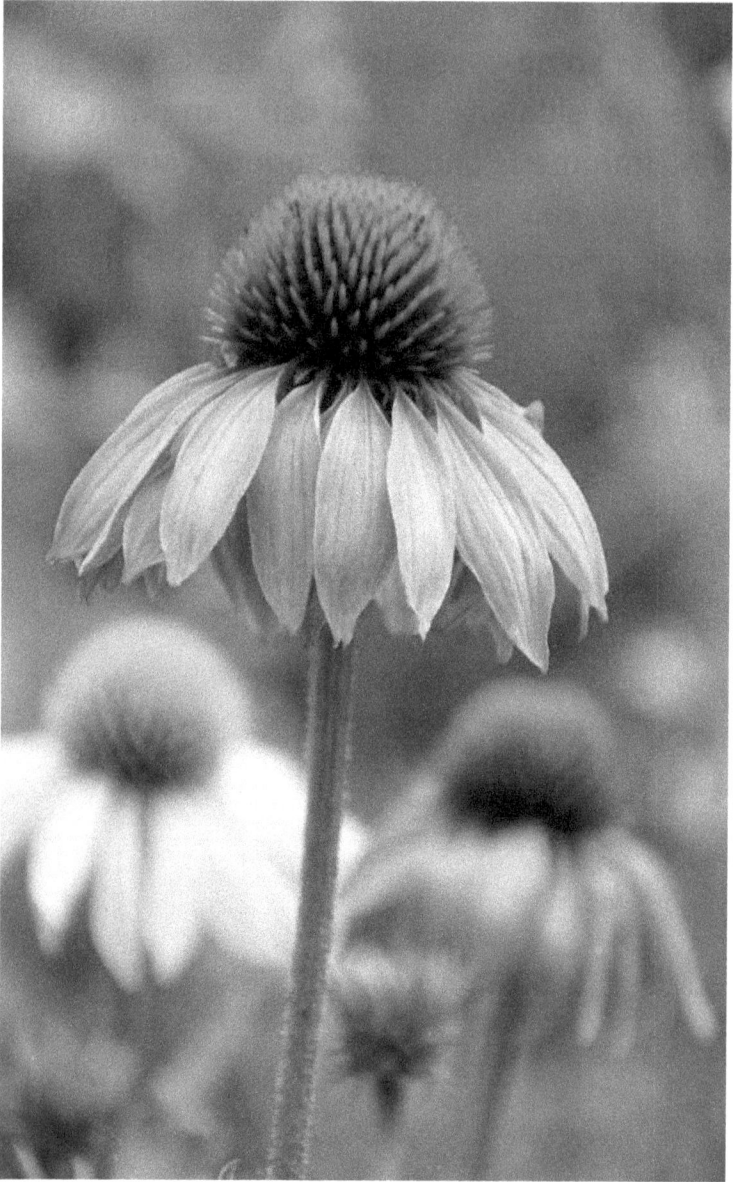

Chapter 3

Natural Remedies for RSV

Herbal remedies for RSV

Respiratory Syncytial Virus (RSV) is a common virus that can cause respiratory infections in people of all ages, but it is particularly dangerous for infants and young children. While there are medications available to treat RSV, many people are turning to herbal remedies as a natural alternative to help prevent and alleviate symptoms associated with the virus.

In this chapter, we will explore some of the most effective herbal remedies for RSV and how they can be incorporated into your daily routine.

One of the most popular herbal remedies for RSV is elderberry. Elderberry is rich in antioxidants and has been shown to have antiviral properties that can help boost the immune system and reduce the severity and duration of respiratory infections.

Elderberry can be taken in the form of syrup, capsules, or teas and is safe for both children and adults. Adding elderberry to your daily routine can help prevent RSV and other respiratory infections.

Another powerful herbal remedy for RSV is licorice root. Licorice root has anti-inflammatory and antiviral properties that can help reduce inflammation in the respiratory tract and fight off viral infections. Licorice root can be taken in the form of tea or capsules and is safe for both children and adults. Incorporating licorice root into your daily routine can help prevent RSV and provide relief from symptoms if you do become infected.

Echinacea is another herbal remedy that can help prevent and alleviate symptoms of RSV. Echinacea has immune-boosting properties that can help strengthen the immune system and fight off viral infections. Echinacea can be taken in the form of tea, capsules, or tinctures and is safe for both children and adults. Adding echinacea to your daily routine can help prevent RSV and reduce the severity of symptoms if you do contract the virus.

In addition to elderberry, licorice root, and echinacea, there are several other herbal remedies that can help prevent and alleviate symptoms of RSV. Some of these include ginger, turmeric, and oregano oil, all of which have antiviral and immune-boosting properties.

It is important to consult with a healthcare provider or herbalist before starting any herbal remedies to ensure they are safe and appropriate for your individual needs.

In conclusion, herbal remedies can be a safe and effective way to prevent and alleviate symptoms of RSV naturally. By incorporating herbs like elderberry, licorice root, and echinacea into your daily routine, you can help boost your immune system and reduce the risk of contracting RSV.

Remember to consult with a healthcare provider before starting any herbal remedies, and always listen to your body and adjust your treatment plan as needed.

Essential oils for RSV prevention

Essential oils have been used for centuries for their medicinal properties, and they can be a powerful tool in preventing respiratory syncytial virus (RSV). RSV is a common respiratory virus that can cause mild cold-like symptoms in healthy adults, but it can be more severe in infants, older adults, and people with weakened immune systems.

By incorporating essential oils into your daily routine, you can help boost your immune system and protect yourself from RSV.

One of the most effective essential oils for preventing RSV is eucalyptus oil. Eucalyptus oil has powerful antiviral properties that can help fight off RSV and other respiratory infections. You can diffuse eucalyptus oil in your home using a diffuser, or apply it topically to your chest and throat to help clear your airways and prevent infection.

Another essential oil that is great for preventing RSV is tea tree oil. Tea tree oil has strong antimicrobial properties that can help kill off viruses and bacteria that cause respiratory infections. You can add a few drops of tea tree oil to a bowl of hot water and inhale the steam to help clear your sinuses and prevent RSV.

Lavender oil is another essential oil that can help prevent RSV. Lavender oil has calming and relaxing properties that can help reduce stress and boost your immune system. By diffusing lavender oil in your home or adding a few drops to a warm bath, you can help support your body's natural defenses against RSV.

Peppermint oil is also a great essential oil for preventing RSV. Peppermint oil has antibacterial and antiviral properties that can help fight off infections and keep your respiratory system healthy. You can add a few drops of peppermint oil to a bowl of hot water and inhale the steam, or apply it topically to your chest and throat to help prevent RSV.

Incorporating essential oils into your daily routine can be a simple and effective way to help prevent RSV. By using oils like eucalyptus, tea tree, lavender, and peppermint, you can boost your immune system, clear your airways, and protect yourself from respiratory infections. Take control of your health and try using essential oils for RSV prevention today.

Vitamins and supplements for RSV prevention

As we continue to explore natural solutions for preventing RSV, it is important to consider the role that vitamins and supplements can play in boosting our immune systems and protecting us from this common respiratory virus. While there is no cure for RSV, taking proactive steps to strengthen our bodies can help reduce the risk of infection and lessen the severity of symptoms if we do become sick.

One key vitamin that has been shown to support immune function is Vitamin C. This powerful antioxidant helps to neutralize harmful pathogens in the body and can reduce the duration and severity of respiratory infections. Incorporating Vitamin C-rich foods like oranges, strawberries, and bell peppers into your diet, or taking a daily supplement, can help keep your immune system strong and resilient against RSV.

Another important vitamin for RSV prevention is Vitamin D. Known as the "sunshine vitamin," Vitamin D plays a crucial role in activating immune defenses and reducing inflammation in the respiratory tract. Spending time outdoors in the sunlight, eating Vitamin D-fortified foods like fatty fish and fortified dairy products, or taking a Vitamin D supplement can all help support your immune system and protect against RSV.

In addition to vitamins, certain supplements can also be beneficial for preventing RSV. Probiotics, for example, have been shown to enhance immune function and reduce the risk of respiratory infections. By promoting a healthy balance of gut bacteria, probiotics can help strengthen the body's defenses against RSV and other viruses.

It is important to consult with a healthcare provider before adding any new vitamins or supplements to your routine, especially if you have underlying health conditions or are taking medications. By incorporating these natural solutions into your daily regimen, you can help boost your immune system and reduce the risk of RSV infection, keeping yourself and your loved ones healthy and protected.

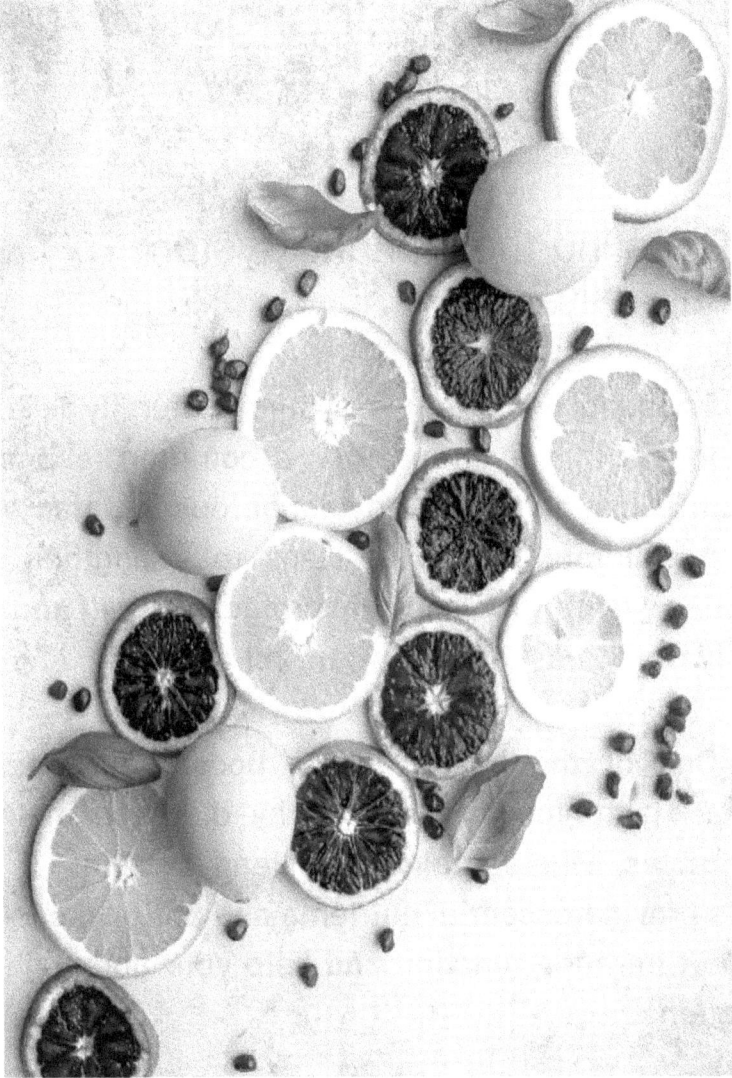

Chapter 4

Lifestyle Changes to Prevent RSV

Boosting the immune system naturally

Boosting the immune system naturally is a key component in preventing RSV, a common respiratory virus that can be particularly dangerous for infants and young children. By taking steps to strengthen your immune system, you can help protect yourself and your family from this potentially harmful virus.

One of the best ways to boost your immune system is to focus on a healthy diet rich in fruits, vegetables, whole grains, and lean proteins. These foods provide essential nutrients and antioxidants that support immune function and help your body fight off infections.

In addition to eating a healthy diet, regular exercise is another important way to boost your immune system naturally. Exercise has been shown to improve immune function and help your body defend against viruses like RSV.

Aim to get at least 30 minutes of moderate exercise most days of the week, such as brisk walking, cycling, or swimming. Not only will exercise strengthen your immune system, but it can also improve your overall health and well-being.

Getting enough sleep is also crucial for a strong immune system. During sleep, your body repairs and regenerates cells, including those involved in your immune response. Aim for 7-9 hours of quality sleep each night to support your immune system and reduce your risk of infections like RSV.

If you have trouble sleeping, try establishing a bedtime routine, avoiding screens before bed, and creating a restful sleep environment.

Stress can weaken your immune system and make you more susceptible to infections like RSV. To reduce stress and support your immune system, try relaxation techniques such as deep breathing, meditation, yoga, or tai chi. These practices can help calm your mind and body, reduce stress hormones, and boost your immune function.

Additionally, finding healthy ways to cope with stress, such as talking to a friend or counselor, can further support your immune system and overall health.

Incorporating immune-boosting herbs and supplements into your daily routine can also help prevent RSV and other viral infections. Some herbs and supplements that have been shown to support immune function include echinacea, elderberry, vitamin C, and zinc. Consult with a healthcare provider before starting any new supplements to ensure they are safe and appropriate for you.

By taking these natural steps to boost your immune system, you can help protect yourself and your family from RSV and other respiratory infections.

Hygiene practices to prevent RSV

Respiratory syncytial virus (RSV) is a common virus that affects the respiratory tract, particularly in young children and older adults. While RSV can be serious and even life-threatening in some cases, there are simple hygiene practices that can help prevent the spread of the virus. By incorporating these practices into your daily routine, you can reduce your risk of contracting RSV and protect those around you.

One of the most important hygiene practices to prevent RSV is frequent handwashing. RSV is primarily spread through respiratory droplets, but it can also be transmitted by touching contaminated surfaces.

By washing your hands regularly with soap and water, especially after coughing, sneezing, or touching your face, you can reduce the likelihood of spreading the virus to others. Encouraging children to wash their hands frequently can also help prevent the spread of RSV in schools and daycare settings.

Another key hygiene practice to prevent RSV is avoiding close contact with sick individuals. If you or someone in your household is experiencing symptoms of RSV, such as coughing, sneezing, or fever, it is important to limit contact with others to prevent the spread of the virus. This may involve staying home from work or school until symptoms improve, as well as avoiding crowded places where RSV may be more easily transmitted.

In addition to handwashing and avoiding close contact with sick individuals, maintaining a clean and sanitary environment can also help prevent the spread of RSV.

Regularly cleaning and disinfecting commonly touched surfaces, such as doorknobs, light switches, and countertops, can help kill any lingering RSV particles and reduce the risk of transmission. Using disinfectant wipes or sprays that are effective against viruses like RSV can provide an added layer of protection for you and your family.

Lastly, practicing good respiratory hygiene can also help prevent the spread of RSV. Covering your mouth and nose with a tissue or your elbow when coughing or sneezing can help prevent respiratory droplets containing the virus from being released into the air. Encouraging others to do the same can help create a culture of respiratory hygiene that can reduce the spread of RSV in your community.

By incorporating these simple hygiene practices into your daily routine, you can help protect yourself and others from RSV and promote a healthier environment for all.

Diet and nutrition for RSV prevention

Diet and nutrition play a crucial role in preventing respiratory syncytial virus (RSV) infections. By maintaining a healthy diet and ensuring proper nutrition, you can boost your immune system and reduce the risk of contracting RSV. In this subchapter, we will explore the foods and nutrients that can help prevent RSV naturally.

One of the key nutrients for preventing RSV is vitamin C. This powerful antioxidant helps to strengthen the immune system and fight off infections. Foods rich in vitamin C include oranges, strawberries, kiwi, and bell peppers. Incorporating these foods into your diet can help to protect against RSV.

Another important nutrient for RSV prevention is vitamin D. Research has shown that vitamin D plays a crucial role in immune function and can help to reduce the risk of respiratory infections. Foods high in vitamin D include fatty fish, eggs, and fortified milk. In addition to dietary sources, spending time outdoors in the sunlight can also help to boost vitamin D levels.

Probiotics are another key component of a healthy diet for RSV prevention. These beneficial bacteria help to support the immune system and protect against infections. Foods rich in probiotics include yogurt, kefir, and sauerkraut. Adding these foods to your diet can help to maintain a healthy gut microbiome and reduce the risk of RSV.

In addition to specific nutrients, it is important to focus on overall dietary patterns for RSV prevention. A diet rich in fruits, vegetables, whole grains, and lean proteins can help to support overall health and immune function. Avoiding processed foods, sugary drinks, and excessive alcohol can also help to prevent RSV.

By following a healthy diet and ensuring proper nutrition, you can strengthen your immune system and reduce the risk of RSV infections. Incorporating foods rich in vitamin C, vitamin D, and probiotics, as well as maintaining a balanced diet, can help to protect against RSV naturally. Making these dietary changes can have a significant impact on your overall health and well-being, helping you to stay healthy and RSV-free.

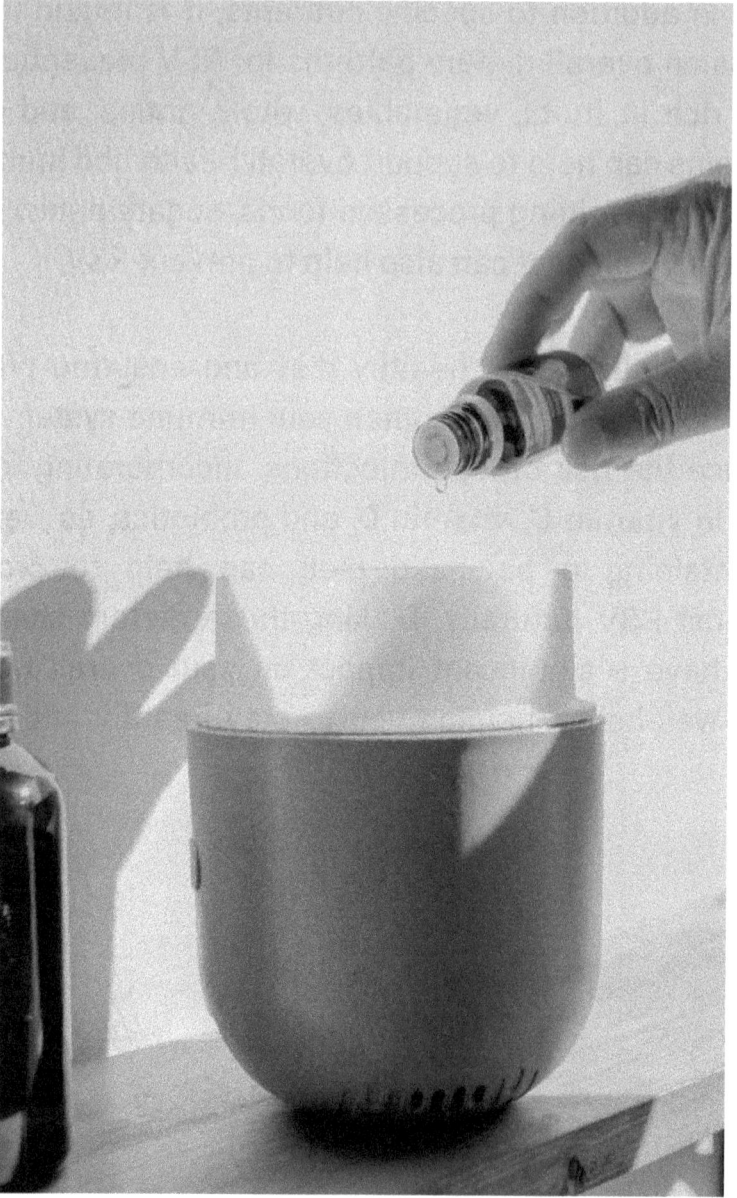

Chapter 5

Home Remedies for RSV Symptoms

Steam therapy for congestion

Steam therapy is a popular and effective natural remedy for relieving congestion caused by respiratory syncytial virus (RSV). By inhaling steam, you can help to loosen mucus in the airways, making it easier to breathe and reducing the symptoms of congestion. Steam therapy is safe and gentle, making it suitable for people of all ages, including infants and children.

To administer steam therapy, simply fill a bowl with hot water and add a few drops of essential oils such as eucalyptus or peppermint. Then, lean over the bowl and inhale the steam for 5-10 minutes. You can also use a humidifier to create a steam-filled environment in your home, which can help to keep airways moist and reduce congestion.

Steam therapy works by helping to open up the airways and reduce inflammation in the respiratory tract. This can help to relieve symptoms such as coughing, wheezing, and difficulty breathing. Steam therapy can also help to soothe irritated nasal passages and reduce the discomfort associated with congestion.

In addition to steam therapy, there are other natural remedies that can help to prevent and relieve congestion caused by RSV. These include staying hydrated, using saline nasal sprays, and using warm compresses on the chest or sinuses. By incorporating these natural remedies into your daily routine, you can help to keep your respiratory system healthy and reduce your risk of developing RSV.

Overall, steam therapy is a simple and effective way to relieve congestion caused by RSV. By inhaling steam, you can help to open up your airways, reduce inflammation, and soothe irritated nasal passages. Incorporating steam therapy into your daily routine, along with other natural remedies, can help to prevent and alleviate the symptoms of RSV, keeping you and your family healthy and happy.

Humidifiers and air purifiers for respiratory health

Humidifiers and air purifiers are essential tools in maintaining respiratory health, especially for those who are concerned about RSV. Humidifiers help to add moisture to the air, which can alleviate symptoms of respiratory illnesses such as RSV. Dry air can irritate the respiratory system and make it more susceptible to infections. By using a humidifier, you can create a more comfortable environment that is less likely to exacerbate respiratory issues.

Air purifiers are another important tool in preventing respiratory illnesses like RSV. These devices work by filtering out harmful particles and pollutants from the air, including dust, pollen, pet dander, and mold spores.

By removing these irritants from the air, air purifiers can help to reduce the risk of respiratory infections and improve overall respiratory health. This is especially important for those who are at higher risk of developing RSV, such as young children, the elderly, and individuals with compromised immune systems.

When choosing a humidifier or air purifier for respiratory health, it is important to consider the size of the room you will be using it in. A humidifier that is too small for the space will not effectively add moisture to the air, while an air purifier that is too small may not be able to filter out all of the harmful particles.

It is also important to regularly clean and maintain these devices to ensure that they are working properly and effectively.

In addition to using humidifiers and air purifiers, there are other natural solutions that can help prevent RSV and maintain respiratory health. These include maintaining good hygiene practices, such as washing hands regularly and avoiding close contact with sick individuals. Eating a healthy diet rich in vitamins and minerals can also help to support a strong immune system and reduce the risk of respiratory infections.

By incorporating humidifiers and air purifiers into your respiratory health routine, along with other natural preventative measures, you can help to protect yourself and your loved ones from respiratory illnesses like RSV.

Taking a proactive approach to respiratory health is key to staying healthy and preventing infections, especially during the cold and flu season when respiratory illnesses are more prevalent.

Natural cough remedies

For those concerned about RSV, it's important to know that there are natural remedies available to help alleviate symptoms of coughing. These remedies can be effective in soothing your throat and reducing the frequency and severity of coughing fits. In this subchapter, we will explore some of the best natural cough remedies that can help you manage your symptoms and prevent the spread of RSV.

One of the most effective natural cough remedies is honey. Honey has been used for centuries as a natural remedy for coughs and sore throats. Its soothing properties help to coat the throat and reduce irritation, leading to less frequent coughing. You can take a spoonful of honey on its own, or mix it with warm water or tea for added relief.

Another natural cough remedy is ginger. Ginger has anti-inflammatory properties that can help reduce inflammation in the throat and airways, leading to less coughing. You can add fresh ginger to hot water or tea, or use ginger essential oil in a diffuser to help alleviate coughing.

Steam inhalation is another effective natural remedy for coughing. Inhaling steam can help to loosen mucus in the airways and reduce coughing. You can simply fill a bowl with hot water and lean over it with a towel over your head to trap the steam, or use a steam inhaler for more targeted relief.

Saltwater gargles are a simple yet effective natural remedy for coughing. Gargling with warm salt water can help to reduce inflammation in the throat and soothe irritation, leading to less coughing. Simply mix a teaspoon of salt in a glass of warm water and gargle for 30 seconds before spitting out.

Finally, staying hydrated is crucial when it comes to managing coughing and preventing the spread of RSV. Drinking plenty of water helps to keep your throat moist and reduce irritation, leading to less frequent coughing. You can also drink herbal teas and warm broths to help soothe your throat and alleviate coughing. By incorporating these natural cough remedies into your routine, you can effectively manage your symptoms and prevent the spread of RSV in a safe and natural way.

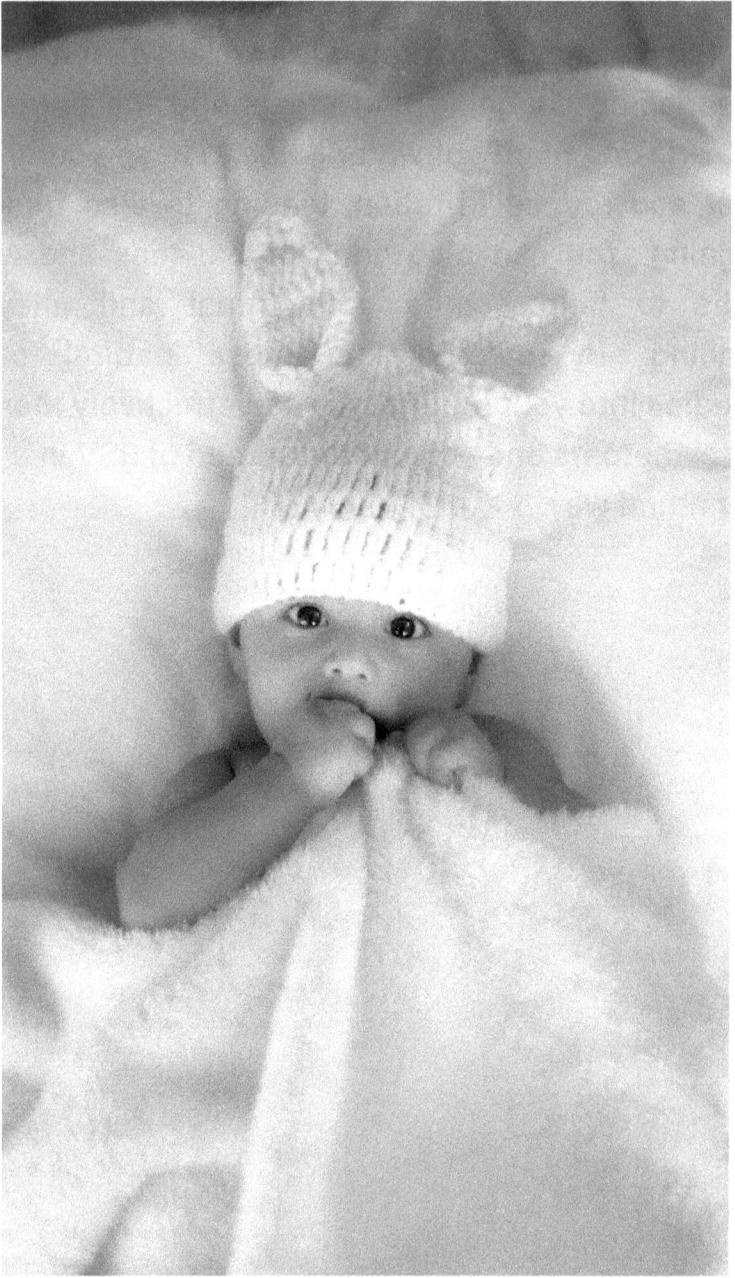

Chapter 6

Preventing RSV in Children

RSV prevention tips for infants

RSV, or respiratory syncytial virus, is a common virus that can affect people of all ages, but it can be particularly dangerous for infants. In this subchapter, we will discuss some tips for preventing RSV in infants naturally. By taking these precautions, you can help protect your little one from this potentially serious illness.

One of the most important things you can do to prevent RSV in infants is to practice good hygiene. This means washing your hands frequently with soap and water, especially before touching your baby or preparing their food.

You should also make sure that anyone who comes into contact with your baby follows these same hygiene practices to reduce the risk of spreading the virus.

Another key tip for preventing RSV in infants is to avoid exposing them to large crowds, especially during peak RSV season, which typically runs from late fall to early spring. By limiting your baby's exposure to germs and viruses in crowded places, you can help reduce their risk of contracting RSV.

It's also important to keep your baby's environment clean and free of germs. This means regularly disinfecting surfaces that your baby touches frequently, such as toys, bottles, and pacifiers. You should also make sure that your baby's bedding and clothing are washed regularly in hot water to kill any germs that may be present.

Finally, it's crucial to ensure that your baby is up to date on their vaccinations, as this can help protect them from RSV and other serious illnesses. Talk to your pediatrician about the recommended vaccination schedule for your baby and make sure to follow it closely. By following these tips and taking proactive measures to prevent RSV in infants, you can help keep your little one healthy and happy.

RSV prevention strategies for toddlers

RSV, or Respiratory Syncytial Virus, is a common respiratory virus that can affect people of all ages, but it is particularly dangerous for toddlers. In this subchapter, we will discuss some key strategies for preventing RSV in toddlers using natural solutions.

One of the most effective ways to prevent RSV in toddlers is to practice good hygiene. This includes washing hands frequently with soap and water, especially before eating or touching the face. Encouraging toddlers to cover their mouths and noses when coughing or sneezing can also help prevent the spread of the virus.

Another important strategy for preventing RSV in toddlers is to ensure they are getting proper nutrition and plenty of rest. A healthy immune system is better equipped to fight off infections, so it is essential to provide toddlers with a balanced diet rich in fruits, vegetables, and whole grains. Making sure they get enough sleep each night can also help support their immune system.

In addition to good hygiene and proper nutrition, there are natural remedies that can help prevent RSV in toddlers. Some parents find that using essential oils, such as eucalyptus or tea tree oil, in a diffuser can help clear the airways and reduce the risk of respiratory infections. Others swear by the benefits of elderberry syrup, which is believed to boost the immune system and ward off viruses.

It is also important to limit toddlers' exposure to others who may be sick. Avoiding crowded places during peak RSV season, which typically runs from late fall to early spring, can help reduce the risk of infection. Encouraging visitors to wash their hands before interacting with your toddler can also help prevent the spread of the virus.

By following these strategies and incorporating natural remedies into your toddler's routine, you can help reduce their risk of contracting RSV. Remember that prevention is key when it comes to protecting your little one from respiratory infections, so be proactive in implementing these strategies to keep them healthy and happy.

RSV prevention for school-aged children

RSV, or respiratory syncytial virus, is a common respiratory virus that can affect people of all ages, but is especially dangerous for young children. In this subchapter, we will discuss ways to prevent RSV in school-aged children using natural solutions for health. By taking proactive steps to protect your child from RSV, you can help them avoid serious illness and potential complications.

One of the most effective ways to prevent RSV in school-aged children is to ensure they practice good hygiene habits. Encourage your child to wash their hands frequently, especially after being in crowded places or touching surfaces that may be contaminated with the virus. By teaching your child proper handwashing techniques, you can help reduce their risk of contracting RSV.

Another important aspect of RSV prevention for school-aged children is to ensure they have a healthy immune system. Make sure your child gets plenty of rest, eats a balanced diet rich in fruits and vegetables, and stays active to boost their immune system.

Additionally, consider incorporating immune-boosting supplements such as vitamin C, zinc, and echinacea into your child's daily routine to help protect them from RSV.

It is also crucial to teach your child about the importance of respiratory etiquette. Encourage them to cover their mouth and nose with a tissue or their elbow when coughing or sneezing to prevent the spread of respiratory droplets that may contain the RSV virus. By instilling these habits in your child, you can help protect them and others from contracting RSV.

Lastly, consider using natural remedies to help prevent RSV in school-aged children. Essential oils such as eucalyptus and tea tree oil have antibacterial and antiviral properties that can help boost your child's immune system and prevent respiratory infections. Additionally, consider using a humidifier in your child's room to keep the air moist, which can help prevent the spread of viruses like RSV. By incorporating these natural solutions into your child's routine, you can help protect them from RSV and other respiratory illnesses.

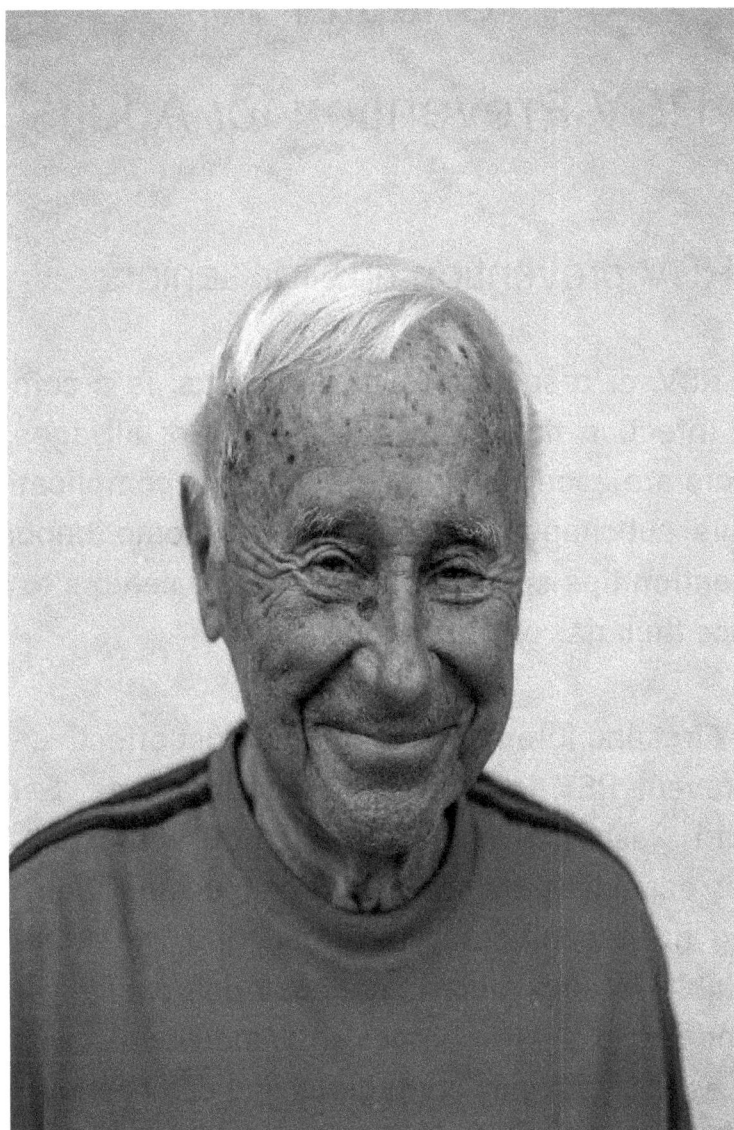

Chapter 7

RSV Prevention for Adults

RSV prevention tips for seniors

RSV, or respiratory syncytial virus, is a common viral infection that can affect people of all ages, but seniors are especially vulnerable to its complications. In this subchapter, we will discuss some important prevention tips specifically tailored for seniors to help reduce their risk of contracting RSV.

First and foremost, one of the most effective ways to prevent RSV is to practice good hygiene. Seniors should wash their hands frequently with soap and water, especially before eating or touching their face. Using hand sanitizer when soap and water are not available is also recommended. Additionally, seniors should avoid close contact with individuals who are sick, as RSV is highly contagious and can easily spread through respiratory droplets.

Another important prevention tip for seniors is to ensure their immune system is strong and healthy. This can be achieved through a balanced diet rich in fruits, vegetables, and whole grains, as well as regular exercise and plenty of rest. Seniors should also consider taking supplements such as vitamin C and zinc to support their immune system and help prevent RSV infection.

Seniors should also make sure to keep their living environment clean and well-ventilated. Regularly disinfecting commonly-touched surfaces such as doorknobs, light switches, and countertops can help reduce the spread of RSV. Using a humidifier in the home can also help keep the air moist, which can prevent the virus from surviving on surfaces for extended periods.

Lastly, seniors should stay up to date on their vaccinations, including the flu vaccine. While the flu vaccine does not protect against RSV specifically, it can help reduce the severity of symptoms and prevent complications that may arise from contracting both viruses simultaneously. By following these prevention tips, seniors can greatly reduce their risk of RSV and stay healthy throughout the year.

RSV prevention strategies for individuals with compromised immune systems

For individuals with compromised immune systems, preventing respiratory syncytial virus (RSV) is especially important. RSV is a common virus that can cause mild cold-like symptoms in healthy individuals, but it can lead to severe respiratory infections in those with weakened immune systems.

In this subchapter, we will discuss some strategies that can help individuals with compromised immune systems reduce their risk of contracting RSV.

One of the most important prevention strategies for individuals with compromised immune systems is to avoid close contact with people who are sick. RSV is highly contagious and can spread through respiratory droplets when an infected person coughs or sneezes. By staying away from sick individuals, those with compromised immune systems can reduce their risk of exposure to the virus.

Another important prevention strategy is to practice good hand hygiene. Regularly washing hands with soap and water for at least 20 seconds can help remove any RSV virus particles that may be on the hands. Using hand sanitizer with at least 60% alcohol is also effective in killing germs and reducing the spread of RSV.

It is also important for individuals with compromised immune systems to avoid touching their face, especially their eyes, nose, and mouth. RSV can enter the body through mucous membranes, so avoiding touching the face can help prevent the virus from entering the body. Additionally, wearing a mask in crowded or high-risk settings can provide an extra layer of protection against RSV.

Staying healthy and maintaining a strong immune system is another key prevention strategy for individuals with compromised immune systems. Eating a balanced diet, getting regular exercise, staying hydrated, and getting enough sleep can all help support the immune system and reduce the risk of infections like RSV.

It is also important for individuals with compromised immune systems to follow their doctor's recommendations for vaccinations and medications that can help prevent infections.

By following these prevention strategies, individuals with compromised immune systems can reduce their risk of contracting RSV and stay healthy. It is important to be proactive in taking steps to prevent infections, especially for those who are more vulnerable to severe illness. With proper precautions and good hygiene practices, individuals with compromised immune systems can protect themselves against RSV and other respiratory infections.

Workplace precautions to prevent RSV transmission

RSV, or respiratory syncytial virus, is a common respiratory virus that can cause serious illness in people of all ages. In the workplace, it is important to take precautions to prevent the spread of RSV and protect yourself and your coworkers from getting sick. By following some simple guidelines, you can help reduce the risk of RSV transmission in your workplace.

One of the most important things you can do to prevent RSV transmission in the workplace is to practice good hand hygiene. Washing your hands frequently with soap and water for at least 20 seconds can help remove any viruses that may be on your hands. Using hand sanitizer with at least 60% alcohol is also effective in killing germs and preventing the spread of RSV. Encourage your coworkers to do the same to help reduce the risk of transmission.

Another key precaution to take in the workplace is to avoid close contact with anyone who is sick. RSV is highly contagious and can be spread through respiratory droplets when an infected person coughs or sneezes.

If a coworker is showing symptoms of RSV, such as a runny nose, cough, or fever, encourage them to stay home until they are no longer contagious. This will help prevent the virus from spreading to others in the workplace.

In addition to practicing good hand hygiene and avoiding close contact with sick coworkers, it is also important to clean and disinfect frequently touched surfaces in the workplace. RSV can survive on surfaces for several hours, so regularly cleaning and disinfecting doorknobs, light switches, keyboards, and other commonly touched surfaces can help prevent the spread of the virus.

Encourage your coworkers to do the same to help keep the workplace clean and germ-free.

If you work in a healthcare setting or other high-risk environment, it may be necessary to wear personal protective equipment, such as masks and gloves, to prevent RSV transmission. These precautions can help protect you and your coworkers from coming into contact with the virus and reduce the risk of getting sick.

Following all workplace guidelines and protocols for infection control can help prevent the spread of RSV and keep everyone safe and healthy.

By taking simple precautions in the workplace, you can help prevent the spread of RSV and protect yourself and your coworkers from getting sick. Practicing good hand hygiene, avoiding close contact with sick coworkers, cleaning and disinfecting frequently touched surfaces, and wearing personal protective equipment when necessary are all important steps in preventing RSV transmission. By working together and following these guidelines, you can create a safer and healthier workplace for everyone.

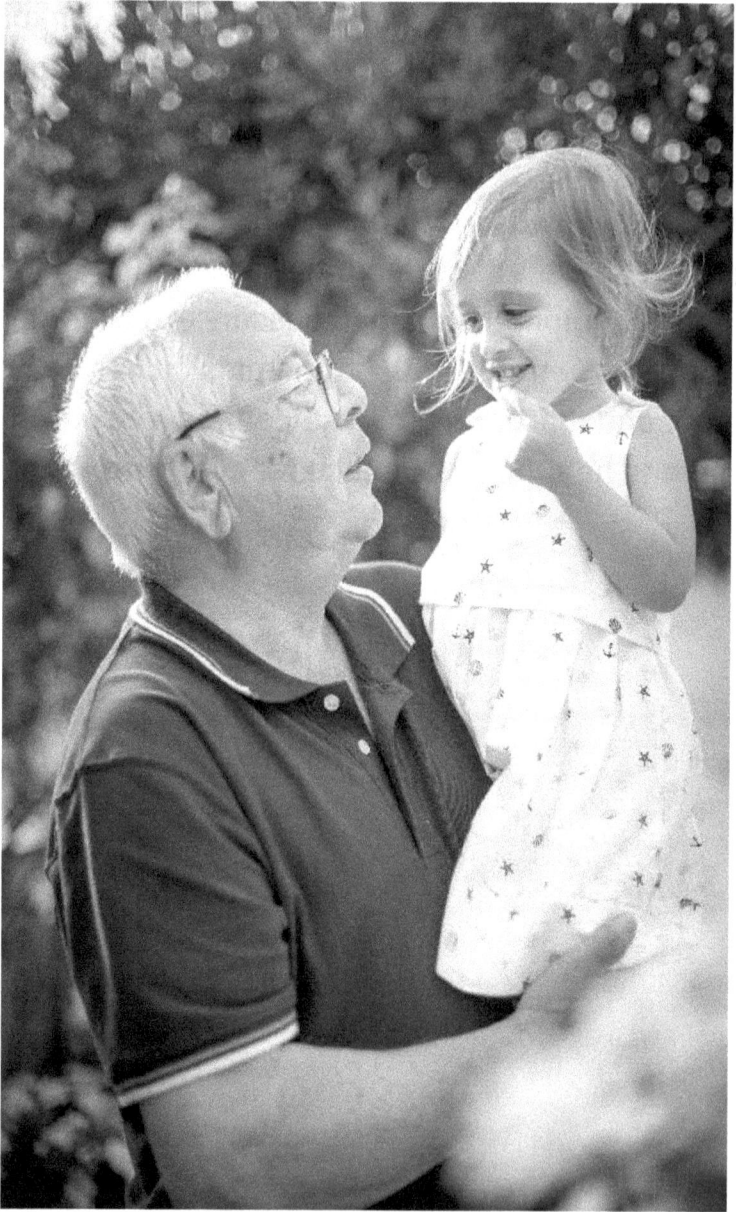

Chapter 8

Conclusion

Recap of natural RSV prevention methods

In this subchapter, we will recap some of the most effective natural methods for preventing respiratory syncytial virus (RSV). RSV is a common virus that affects the respiratory system, particularly in young children and the elderly. By taking proactive steps to boost your immune system and maintain good hygiene practices, you can reduce your risk of contracting RSV and protect yourself and your loved ones from this potentially serious illness.

One of the most important ways to prevent RSV naturally is to focus on boosting your immune system. Eating a healthy diet rich in fruits, vegetables, and whole grains can help provide your body with the vitamins and nutrients it needs to fight off infections. Additionally, getting regular exercise, staying hydrated, and getting enough sleep are all important factors in maintaining a strong immune system.

Another key aspect of natural RSV prevention is practicing good hygiene. Washing your hands regularly with soap and water, especially before eating or touching your face, can help prevent the spread of RSV and other viruses. Avoiding close contact with sick individuals and staying home when you are feeling unwell can also help reduce your risk of contracting RSV.

In addition to these general preventative measures, there are also specific natural remedies that can help boost your immune system and protect against RSV. Herbal supplements like echinacea, elderberry, and astragalus have been shown to have immune-boosting properties and may help prevent respiratory infections.

Essential oils like tea tree, eucalyptus, and peppermint can also be used to help clear congestion and support respiratory health.

By incorporating these natural RSV prevention methods into your daily routine, you can take proactive steps to protect yourself and your loved ones from this common virus.

Remember to focus on boosting your immune system, practicing good hygiene, and using natural remedies to support respiratory health. With a little effort and diligence, you can reduce your risk of contracting RSV and stay healthy all year round.

Creating a personalized RSV prevention plan

RSV, or respiratory syncytial virus, is a common virus that can cause respiratory infections in people of all ages, but it is especially dangerous for infants and young children. In order to protect yourself and your loved ones from RSV, it is important to create a personalized prevention plan that takes into account your specific risk factors and lifestyle choices.

The first step in creating a personalized RSV prevention plan is to assess your individual risk factors. If you have young children, work in a healthcare setting, or have a weakened immune system, you may be at a higher risk of contracting RSV. By identifying these risk factors, you can take proactive steps to reduce your chances of getting sick.

One of the most effective ways to prevent RSV is to practice good hygiene. This includes washing your hands frequently with soap and water, avoiding close contact with sick individuals, and disinfecting commonly-touched surfaces in your home or workplace. By incorporating these simple habits into your daily routine, you can significantly reduce your risk of exposure to RSV.

In addition to practicing good hygiene, it is also important to support your immune system through healthy lifestyle choices. Eating a balanced diet rich in fruits and vegetables, getting regular exercise, and managing stress can all help to strengthen your body's natural defenses against respiratory infections like RSV. By taking care of your overall health, you can reduce your susceptibility to illness and improve your chances of staying well.

Finally, it is important to stay informed about the latest developments in RSV prevention and treatment. By staying up-to-date on current recommendations from healthcare professionals and public health authorities, you can make informed decisions about how to protect yourself and your loved ones from RSV.

By combining these strategies into a personalized prevention plan, you can take control of your health and reduce your risk of contracting respiratory infections like RSV.

Resources for further information on RSV prevention

If you are looking for more information on how to prevent RSV naturally, there are several resources available to help you in your journey towards better health. Below are some resources that you may find useful:

1. The Centers for Disease Control and Prevention (CDC) website is a great place to start when looking for information on RSV prevention. The CDC offers detailed information on the symptoms of RSV, how it spreads, and what steps you can take to protect yourself and your family from this virus.

2. The National Institute of Allergy and Infectious Diseases (NIAID) also provides valuable information on RSV prevention. Their website offers up-to-date research on the virus, as well as tips on how to reduce your risk of infection and keep your immune system strong.

3. The World Health Organization (WHO) is another excellent resource for information on RSV prevention. The WHO website offers global statistics on RSV cases, as well as recommendations for preventing the spread of the virus in different communities.

4. The American Academy of Pediatrics (AAP) is a trusted source for information on child health and wellness. Their website offers tips for parents on how to protect their children from RSV, as well as resources for healthcare providers on diagnosing and treating the virus.

5. Finally, books such as "The RSV Prevention Handbook: Natural Solutions for Health" can be a valuable resource for those looking to learn more about natural ways to prevent RSV. This book offers practical advice on boosting your immune system, maintaining good hygiene practices, and creating a healthy living environment to reduce your risk of infection.

By utilizing these resources, you can empower yourself with the knowledge and tools needed to protect yourself and your loved ones from RSV. Remember, prevention is key when it comes to staying healthy, so take the time to educate yourself and take proactive steps to reduce your risk of infection.

Author Notes & Acknowledgments

First and foremost, I would like to express my deepest gratitude to the people who inspired and supported me throughout the journey of writing this book. This project would not have been possible without their unwavering belief in me and their invaluable contributions.

To my wife, thank you for your constant encouragement and understanding. Your love and support have been my anchor during the challenging times of researching and writing this book. Your belief in my ability to make a difference in people's lives has been my driving force.

I would also like to disclose that this book contains some renewed artificial intelligence-generated content. I really appreciate very recent technological innovation by outstanding scientists and of course our reader's understanding.

Lastly, I want to express my deepest gratitude to the readers of this book. I sincerely hope the strategies and methods outlined within these pages will provide you with the knowledge and tools needed to truly make your life much better. Your commitment to seeking any good solutions and willingness to explore multiple methods is commendable.

Author Bio

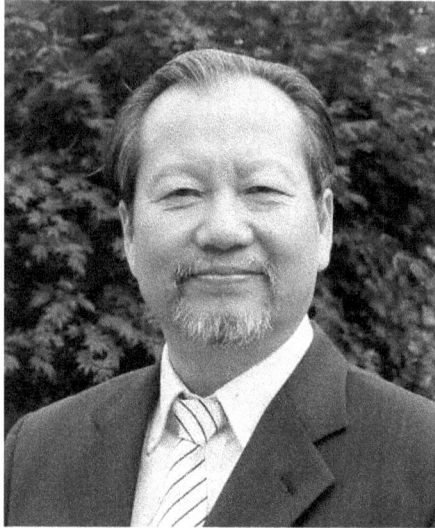

Johnson Wu earned his MD in 1982. With over 40 years of clinical experience, he has worked in hospitals in Zhejiang and Shanghai, China, as well as the Royal Marsden Hospital (part of Imperial College) in London, UK.

Upon the recommendation of Sir Aaron Klug, the president of The Royal Society and a Nobel Prize winner in Chemistry, Dr. Wu was honorably awarded a British Royal Society Fellowship. He has published medical books and articles in seven countries and currently practices medicine in Canada.

www.ingramcontent.com/pod-product-compliance
Lightning Source LLC
Chambersburg PA
CBHW060257030426
42335CB00014B/1736